The Yogic Diet

By Dan Lexow

Imprint:

Daniel Lexow

Wilhelm-Külz-Straße 22

17033 Neubrandenburg

www.danlexow.de

THE YOGIC DIET

DAN LEXOW

Table of contents

Part V: Integrating the yogic diet into daily life

Bonus

Conclusion

Introduction

Welcome to the yogic diet

Welcome to the transformative journey of the yogic diet, an ancient practice rooted in the timeless traditions of ayurveda and yoga. This diet is not just a means to nourish your body, but a holistic approach to harmonize your mind, body, and spirit. The yogic diet transcends the ordinary, aiming to cultivate a balanced life filled with vitality, clarity, and spiritual growth. Whether you are a seasoned yogi or a curious beginner, embracing the yogic diet can lead to profound changes in your overall well-being.

The yogic diet emphasizes foods that are pure, simple, and natural, aligning with the principles of sattva—purity and lightness. This dietary approach is designed to enhance your yoga practice, support your meditation, and improve your physical health. By choosing foods that are fresh, organic, and minimally processed, you can foster a deeper connection with nature and your inner self.

The philosophy behind yogic eating

The philosophy of yogic eating is deeply intertwined with the teachings of yoga and Ayurveda, which date back thousands of years. These ancient systems recognize the powerful connection between what we eat and our mental, physical, and spiritual states. The yogic diet categorizes foods into three main types: sattvic (pure and harmonious), rajasic (stimulating and active), and tamasic (dull and inert).

Sattvic foods: These are the foundation of the yogic diet. Sattvic foods are fresh, organic, and minimally processed. They include fruits, vegetables, whole grains, nuts, seeds, and dairy products like milk and ghee. These foods are believed to enhance vitality, mental clarity, and spiritual growth. They promote calmness, focus, and a balanced state of mind.

Rajasic foods: These foods are stimulating and can lead to restlessness and agitation if consumed in excess. Examples include spicy foods, caffeine, and processed snacks. While they can provide quick energy and excitement, they are best consumed in moderation to maintain mental equilibrium and avoid overstimulation.

Tamasic foods: These foods are heavy, dull, and can promote lethargy and confusion. Tamasic foods include meat, alcohol, and overly processed or stale items. They are thought to hinder spiritual progress and should be minimized or avoided for optimal health and clarity.

The underlying principle of the yogic diet is to cultivate a sattvic lifestyle, which fosters purity, peace, and balance. This approach not only supports your physical health but also enhances your mental clarity and spiritual well-being.

Benefits of a yogic diet for mind, body, and soul

The benefits of a yogic diet are manifold, extending beyond physical nourishment to enrich your mental and spiritual life. Here are some of the key benefits:

Physical health

1. **Improved figestion:** Sattvic foods are easy to digest and help maintain a healthy digestive system. They prevent digestive issues like bloating, constipation, and indigestion.

2. **Enhanced immunity:** The nutrients in sattvic foods boost the immune system, helping your body fight off illnesses and infections more effectively.

3. **Sustained energy levels:** Unlike the quick highs and crashes associated with processed foods and sugars, sattvic foods provide steady, sustained energy throughout the day.

4. **Weight management:** The natural, unprocessed nature of sattvic foods supports healthy weight management without the need for restrictive diets.

Mental Clarity

1. **Increased focus:** Sattvic foods promote mental clarity and concentration, essential for effective meditation and mindfulness practices.

2. **Emotional stability:** A diet rich in sattvic foods helps stabilize mood swings and reduces anxiety and stress.

3. **Better sleep:** The calming effects of sattvic foods contribute to improved sleep quality and regular sleep patterns.

Spiritual Growth

1. **Deepened meditation:** A sattvic diet supports deeper, more effective meditation by promoting mental calmness and focus.

2. **Enhanced mindfulness:** Mindful eating practices encourage a greater connection with your food, fostering gratitude and awareness in everyday life.

3. **Spiritual connection:** By aligning your diet with the principles of sattva, you cultivate a lifestyle that supports your spiritual journey and deepens your connection to your higher self.

A personal journey: how I discovered the yogic diet

My journey with the yogic diet began as a quest for better health and a deeper spiritual connection. As someone who had struggled with various health issues and stress, I was drawn to the holistic approach of yoga and Ayurveda. Initially, I experimented with different diets, searching for one that resonated with my body and mind.

It wasn't until I immersed myself in the study of the yogic diet that I began to see profound changes. By gradually incorporating sattvic foods and mindful eating practices, I experienced improved digestion, increased energy, and a calmer, more focused mind. My yoga practice deepened, and my meditation sessions became more fulfilling.

One of the most significant transformations was my relationship with food. Instead of viewing eating as a mere necessity or source of pleasure, I began to see it as a sacred ritual. Each meal became an opportunity to nourish not just my body, but my mind and spirit as well. This shift in perspective brought a sense of peace and gratitude into my daily life.

The journey was not without challenges. There were times when cravings for rajasic and tamasic foods resurfaced, and social situations made it difficult to stick to a sattvic diet. However, with perseverance and support from my yoga community, I learned to navigate these obstacles and stay committed to my path.

This book is a culmination of my experiences, research, and the wisdom of ancient traditions. It is designed to guide you on your journey toward holistic well-being, providing practical advice, delicious recipes, and insights into the transformative power of the yogic diet. Whether you are new to yoga or a seasoned practitioner, this book will help you cultivate a balanced, healthy, and spiritually fulfilling life.

Conclusion

The yogic diet is more than a set of dietary guidelines; it is a holistic approach to living that fosters physical health, mental clarity, and spiritual growth. By embracing the principles of sattva and incorporating mindful eating practices, you can transform your relationship with food and enhance your overall well-being. This introduction sets the stage for a deeper exploration of the yogic diet, its foundations, nutritional essentials, fasting practices, and practical tips for integrating it into your daily life. Welcome to the journey of a lifetime, one meal at a time.

Part I: Foundations of the yogic diet

The principles of yogic eating

The principles of yogic eating are deeply rooted in the philosophy of yoga and Ayurveda, emphasizing the connection between food, mind, and spirit. These principles are designed to promote purity, balance, and harmony, which are essential for physical health, mental clarity, and spiritual growth. By understanding and applying these principles, you can cultivate a diet that supports your overall well-being and enhances your yoga practice.

Sattvic, rajasic, and tamasic foods

Sattvic foods

Sattvic foods are considered pure, fresh, and natural. They are believed to enhance vitality, mental clarity, and spiritual growth. These foods are light, easy to digest, and promote a calm and focused mind. Examples of sattvic foods include:

- **Fruits and vegetables**: Fresh, seasonal, and preferably organic.

- **Whole grains**: Brown rice, quinoa, barley, and oats.

- **Nuts and seeds**: Almonds, walnuts, sunflower seeds, and flaxseeds.

- **Dairy products**: Milk, ghee (clarified butter), and homemade yogurt.

- **Legumes and beans**: Lentils, chickpeas, and mung beans.

- **Herbs and spices**: Mild spices like turmeric, coriander, and basil.

- **Natural sweeteners**: Honey and jaggery (unrefined cane sugar).

Sattvic foods are known for their nourishing and calming properties. They provide the necessary nutrients for the body while keeping the mind serene and focused, which is essential for deepening one's yoga and meditation practices .

Rajasic foods

Rajasic foods are stimulating and can lead to restlessness and agitation. While they can provide energy and excitement, they are best consumed in moderation to maintain mental equilibrium and avoid overstimulation. Examples of rajasic foods include:

- **Spicy foods**: Hot peppers, garlic, onions, and excessive use of strong spices.

- **Caffeinated beverages**: Coffee, black tea, and energy drinks.

- **Processed foods**: Packaged snacks, fast food, and foods with artificial additives.

- **Refined sugars**: White sugar, sugary snacks, and desserts.

- • **Fermented foods**: Pickles, vinegar, and certain aged cheeses.

Consuming too many rajasic foods can lead to hyperactivity, irritability, and a scattered mind. It is important to balance these foods with sattvic choices to maintain mental and emotional stability .

Tamasic foods

Tamasic foods are heavy, dull, and promote lethargy and confusion. These foods are considered detrimental to both physical and mental health as they can slow down bodily functions and cloud the mind. Examples of tamasic foods include:

- • **Meat and fish**: All types of animal flesh.

- • **Alcohol and recreational drugs**: Substances that dull the mind and senses.

- • **Stale and overripe foods**: Foods that are past their prime and lack freshness.

- • **Highly processed foods**: Foods with artificial preservatives, flavors, and long shelf lives.

- • **Excessively oily or fried foods**: Foods cooked in heavy oils and fats.

Tamasic foods are thought to drain energy, create heaviness in the body, and impede spiritual progress. Minimizing these foods helps maintain vitality and mental clarity .

The importance of balance and harmony

Achieving balance and harmony in your diet is essential for maintaining overall well-being. The yogic diet emphasizes the importance of consuming primarily sattvic foods, while occasionally incorporating rajasic foods for energy and avoiding tamasic foods to prevent lethargy and mental dullness.

1. **Balance in variety**: Incorporate a diverse range of foods to ensure you receive all essential nutrients. Each meal should include a mix of carbohydrates, proteins, and fats, along with plenty of fruits and vegetables.

2. **Mindful eating**: Practice mindfulness during meals by eating slowly, savoring each bite, and being fully present. This enhances digestion, allows you to enjoy your food more, and helps you listen to your body's hunger and satiety signals.

3. **Seasonal eating**: Align your diet with the seasons to take advantage of fresh, locally grown produce. Seasonal foods are more nutritious and support the body's natural rhythms and needs.

4. **Moderation**: Avoid overeating and consuming foods that are too heavy or stimulating. Moderation ensures that your diet supports a balanced state of mind and body.

By adhering to these principles, you can create a diet that supports your physical health, mental clarity, and spiritual growth, ultimately leading to a more harmonious and fulfilling life .

Historical and Cultural Background

The yogic diet has its origins in the ancient Indian traditions of Ayurveda and yoga. Ayurveda, which means "science of life," is a holistic system of medicine that emphasizes the balance of the mind, body, and spirit through diet, lifestyle, and herbal remedies. Yoga, on the other hand, is a spiritual practice that seeks to unite the individual soul with the universal consciousness through physical postures, breath control, meditation, and ethical living.

Ancient Texts and Teachings:
The principles of the yogic diet are derived from ancient scriptures such as the Vedas, Upanishads, Bhagavad Gita, and the Yoga Sutras of Patanjali. These texts highlight the importance of purity, non-violence (ahimsa), and self-discipline in one's diet and lifestyle.

Ayurvedic Principles:
Ayurveda categorizes individuals into three doshas (constitutional types) - Vata, Pitta, and Kapha. Each dosha has unique dietary needs and imbalances that can be corrected through specific foods and lifestyle practices. The yogic diet aligns with Ayurvedic principles by promoting foods that balance the doshas and support overall health.

Cultural Practices:
In traditional Indian culture, food is considered sacred and is often prepared with great care and intention. Meals are seen as offerings to the divine and are consumed with gratitude and mindfulness. This cultural reverence for food is reflected in the yogic diet, which emphasizes the spiritual and energetic qualities of what we eat.

Modern Adaptations:
Today, the yogic diet is embraced by people worldwide who seek to improve their health, deepen their yoga practice, and cultivate a more mindful and conscious way of living. Modern adaptations of the yogic diet include incorporating global ingredients and recipes that align with the principles of sattva, balance, and harmony .

By understanding the historical and cultural background of the yogic diet, you can appreciate the depth and wisdom of this ancient practice and its relevance in today's world. The following chapters will delve deeper into the practical aspects of adopting a yogic diet, including nutritional essentials, meal planning, and fasting practices.

The yogic lifestyle

Integrating diet with yoga practice

The yogic lifestyle is a holistic approach that extends beyond the physical practice of yoga to include diet, mindfulness, and conscious living. Integrating a yogic diet with your yoga practice can enhance both physical and mental well-being, creating a balanced and harmonious life. Here's how you can seamlessly integrate diet with yoga practice:

Synergy of food and asanas

The foods you consume directly affect your energy levels, flexibility, and overall performance during yoga practice. Sattvic foods, known for their purity and balance, provide sustained energy without causing heaviness or lethargy. This allows you to perform asanas (yoga postures) with greater ease and stability.

1. **Pre-Yoga nutrition**: Eating a light meal or snack 2 hours before practice can provide the necessary energy. Opt for fruits, smoothies, or a small serving of nuts and seeds.

2. **Post-Yoga nutrition**: After practice, focus on replenishing nutrients with a balanced meal that includes proteins, healthy fats, and carbohydrates. A vegetable-rich salad with quinoa or a bowl of lentil soup can be ideal.

Timing and mindfulness

Eating at the right times and in the right way is crucial in a yogic lifestyle. Practicing mindful eating, where you are fully present and aware of your food, enhances digestion and absorption of nutrients.

1. **Regular meal times**: Establish a routine with regular meal times to align your body's internal clock with natural rhythms, supporting optimal digestion and energy levels.

2. **Mindful eating**: Avoid distractions during meals. Focus on the taste, texture, and aroma of your food. Chew slowly and thoroughly, allowing your body to register fullness and satisfaction.

Yoga and detoxification

Certain yoga practices, such as twists and inversions, help stimulate the digestive system and support detoxification. A diet rich in sattvic foods complements these practices by aiding in the natural detoxification processes of the body.

1. **Hydration**: Drink plenty of water throughout the day to support digestion and detoxification. Herbal teas and coconut water are also beneficial.

2. **Detoxifying foods**: Include foods like leafy greens, fresh fruits, and herbs such as cilantro and mint, which aid in cleansing the body.

Mindful eating and conscious living

Mindful eating and conscious living are integral components of the yogic lifestyle. These practices foster a deeper connection with your body, your food, and the environment.

Principles of mindful eating

Mindful eating involves being fully present during meals, paying attention to the sensory experience of eating, and recognizing the physical and emotional cues related to hunger and satiety.

1. **Awareness**: Be aware of what you are eating, why you are eating, and how the food makes you feel. This awareness helps you make healthier choices and avoid overeating.

2. **Gratitude**: Cultivate a sense of gratitude for the food you consume. Acknowledge the effort and resources involved in bringing the food to your plate.

3. **Intuition**: Listen to your body's hunger and fullness signals. Eat when you are hungry and stop when you are satisfied.

Conscious living

Conscious living extends beyond the plate, encompassing all aspects of life. It involves making intentional choices that align with your values and promote overall well-being.

1. **Sustainability**: Choose foods that are sustainably sourced and produced. Support local farmers and opt for organic produce to reduce your environmental impact.

2. **Minimalism**: Simplify your life by focusing on what truly matters. This includes decluttering your space, reducing waste, and living with intention.

3. **Mindfulness practices**: Incorporate mindfulness into daily activities, such as walking, cleaning, or even brushing your teeth. Being present in each moment enhances your overall quality of life.

Common misconceptions about the yogic diet

Despite its many benefits, the yogic diet is often misunderstood. Here are some common misconceptions and the truths behind them.

Misconception 1: The yogic diet is strictly vegetarian

Truth:
While traditional yogic diets emphasize vegetarianism due to the principle of ahimsa (non-violence), they can be adapted to individual needs.

The focus is on consuming sattvic foods, which can include dairy products like milk and ghee, but it's not strictly limited to vegetarianism. Some practitioners may include ethically sourced animal products in moderation.

Misconception 2: The yogic diet is bland and restrictive

Truth:
The yogic diet includes a wide variety of delicious and nutritious foods. From vibrant fruits and vegetables to flavorful herbs and spices, the diet is anything but bland. Sattvic recipes can be incredibly diverse and satisfying, offering a range of flavors and textures.

Misconception 3: The yogic diet is only for yogis

Truth:
The benefits of the yogic diet extend to anyone seeking a balanced, healthy lifestyle. Its principles can enhance overall well-being, regardless of whether one practices yoga. The emphasis on fresh, natural, and minimally processed foods supports optimal health for everyone.

Misconception 4: It requires expensive, exotic ingredients

Truth:
While some ingredients like certain herbs and superfoods may seem exotic, the core of the yogic diet consists of simple, easily accessible foods. Fresh fruits, vegetables, whole grains, nuts, and seeds are widely available and affordable. The diet encourages local and seasonal produce, which can be cost-effective and environmentally friendly.

Misconception 5: It's hard to follow in modern life

Truth:
With some planning and mindfulness, the yogic diet can be easily integrated into a modern lifestyle. Meal prepping, mindful eating, and making conscious choices about food sourcing can make adherence to the diet manageable and rewarding. The principles of the yogic diet are flexible and can be adapted to fit various lifestyles and dietary needs.

By understanding and embracing the principles of the yogic diet, you can create a lifestyle that supports not only your physical health but also your mental clarity and spiritual growth. This holistic approach to eating and living fosters a deeper connection with yourself and the world around you, paving the way for a balanced and fulfilling life.

Part II: Yogic Nutrition Essentials

Understanding sattvic foods

Sattvic foods form the cornerstone of the yogic diet, promoting physical health, mental clarity, and spiritual growth. These foods are characterized by their purity, simplicity, and natural qualities, which align with the principles of sattva (purity and harmony). Understanding what constitutes sattvic foods and their health benefits can help you make mindful dietary choices that support your overall well-being.

What are sattvic foods?

Sattvic foods are fresh, natural, and minimally processed, reflecting the qualities of lightness, balance, and purity. They are believed to increase prana (life force) and enhance the mind's clarity and calmness. Here are the main categories of sattvic foods:

Fresh fruits and vegetables

Fruits: Apples, bananas, berries, citrus fruits, grapes, and melons. These fruits are rich in vitamins, minerals, and antioxidants, providing essential nutrients for overall health.

Vegetables: Leafy greens (spinach, kale), root vegetables (carrots, beets), and cruciferous vegetables (broccoli, cauliflower). These vegetables are high in fiber, vitamins, and minerals, supporting digestion and detoxification.

Whole grains

Whole grains such as brown rice, quinoa, barley, and oats are staples in a sattvic diet. These grains are unprocessed and rich in complex carbohydrates, providing sustained energy and supporting digestive health.

Legumes and beans

Legumes and beans, including lentils, chickpeas, and mung beans, are excellent sources of plant-based protein and fiber. They are easy to digest and help maintain balanced blood sugar levels.

Nuts and seeds

Nuts (almonds, walnuts) and seeds (flaxseeds, chia seeds) are nutrient-dense foods that provide healthy fats, protein, and essential minerals. They support brain health, cardiovascular function, and overall vitality.

Dairy products

Dairy products such as milk, ghee (clarified butter), and homemade yogurt are considered sattvic when sourced from ethically treated animals and consumed in moderation. They provide calcium, protein, and beneficial probiotics for gut health.

Herbs and spices

Mild herbs and spices like turmeric, ginger, basil, coriander, and cumin enhance the flavor of foods while offering various health benefits, such as anti-inflammatory and antioxidant properties.

Natural sweeteners

Natural sweeteners like honey and jaggery (unrefined cane sugar) are used in moderation to sweeten foods without the harmful effects of refined sugar. They provide essential nutrients and support energy levels.

Creating balanced meals

Creating balanced meals is a fundamental aspect of the yogic diet, ensuring that your body receives all the essential nutrients it needs to thrive. A balanced meal includes a variety of foods from different food groups, providing carbohydrates, proteins, fats, vitamins, and minerals. Here's a comprehensive guide to creating balanced meals, focusing on the essential nutrients and practical meal planning tips to help you maintain a sattvic lifestyle.

Essential nutrients for a yogic diet

A well-rounded yogic diet includes all the essential nutrients your body needs for optimal health. Here are the key nutrients and their sources within a sattvic diet:

Carbohydrates

Carbohydrates are the body's primary source of energy. Complex carbohydrates, found in whole grains and vegetables, provide sustained energy and support digestive health.

Sources:

- Whole grains: Brown rice, quinoa, millet, barley, and oats.

- Vegetables: Sweet potatoes, carrots, beets, and leafy greens.

Proteins

Proteins are crucial for building and repairing tissues, supporting immune function, and maintaining muscle mass. Plant-based proteins are a staple in the yogic diet.

Sources:

- Legumes: Lentils, chickpeas, black beans, and mung beans.

- Nuts and seeds: Almonds, walnuts, chia seeds, and flaxseeds.

- Dairy: Milk, yogurt, and ghee (for those who include dairy in their diet).

Fats

Healthy fats are essential for brain function, hormone production, and nutrient absorption. The yogic diet includes sources of unsaturated fats and omega-3 fatty acids.

Sources:

- Nuts and seeds: Almonds, walnuts, sunflower seeds, and hemp seeds.

- Oils: Olive oil, coconut oil, and sesame oil.

- Dairy: Ghee and butter (from ethically sourced, grass-fed animals).

Vitamins and minerals

Vitamins and minerals are vital for numerous bodily functions, including immune response, bone health, and energy production. A variety of fruits, vegetables, and nuts ensure adequate intake.

Sources:

- Fruits: Berries, oranges, apples, bananas, and grapes.

- Vegetables: Leafy greens (spinach, kale), cruciferous vegetables (broccoli, cauliflower), and root vegetables (carrots, beets).

- Nuts and seeds: Almonds (vitamin E), sunflower seeds (selenium), and chia seeds (calcium).

Meal planning and preparation tips

Effective meal planning and preparation are key to maintaining a balanced and nutritious yogic diet. Here are some practical tips to help you plan and prepare your meals:

Plan ahead

Planning your meals in advance ensures that you have the necessary ingredients on hand and helps you avoid impulsive, less healthy choices.

1. **Weekly meal plan**: Create a weekly meal plan that includes breakfast, lunch, dinner, and snacks. Focus on incorporating a variety of sattvic foods to cover all essential nutrients.

2. **Grocery list**: Based on your meal plan, make a detailed grocery list to ensure you have everything you need. This helps you stay organized and avoid unnecessary purchases.

Batch cooking

Batch cooking involves preparing larger quantities of food in advance, which can be stored and used throughout the week. This saves time and ensures you always have healthy meals ready.

1. **Cook staples in bulk**: Prepare staples like brown rice, quinoa, lentils, and beans in large quantities. Store them in the refrigerator or freezer for quick meal assembly.

2. **Prep vegetables**: Wash, chop, and store vegetables in airtight containers. This makes it easy to add them to salads, stir-fries, and soups.

Simple and nutritious recipes

Focus on simple, wholesome recipes that highlight the natural flavors of sattvic foods. Here are some ideas for each meal:

Breakfast:

- **Oatmeal with fresh fruits and nuts**: Cook oats with almond milk and top with fresh berries, sliced banana, and a sprinkle of chia seeds.

- **Sattvic smoothie bowl**: Blend spinach, banana, frozen berries, and almond milk. Top with sliced almonds and coconut flakes.

Lunch:

- **Quinoa and vegetable salad**: Mix cooked quinoa with chopped cucumber, cherry tomatoes, bell peppers, and parsley. Dress with olive oil and lemon juice.

- **Lentil and spinach soup**: Sauté onion and garlic, add lentils, vegetable broth, and spices. Simmer until lentils are tender, then stir in fresh spinach.

Dinner:

- **Stir-fried vegetables with tofu**: Sauté tofu cubes with broccoli, bell peppers, and carrots in sesame oil. Season with soy sauce and sesame seeds. Serve over brown rice.

- **Stuffed bell peppers**: Fill bell peppers with a mixture of quinoa, black beans, corn, and spices. Bake until peppers are tender.

Snacks:

- **Fresh fruit salad**: Combine diced pineapple, mango, and blueberries. Garnish with mint leaves.

- **Almond and date energy balls**: Blend almonds, dates, cocoa powder, and coconut oil. Roll into small balls and refrigerate.

Mindful eating

Practice mindful eating by being fully present during meals.
Chew slowly, savor each bite, and appreciate the flavors and
textures of your food. This not only enhances digestion but
also helps you tune into your body's hunger and satiety
signals.

By incorporating these tips into your routine, you can create
balanced meals that support your physical health, mental
clarity, and spiritual growth. Meal planning and mindful
preparation ensure that you stay committed to the
principles of the yogic diet, fostering a harmonious and
fulfilling lifestyle.

Part III: Fasting practices in yogic tradition

Intermittent fasting in yoga

Fasting has been an integral part of various spiritual traditions, including yoga. It is considered a powerful tool for detoxification, spiritual growth, and self-discipline. Among the various fasting methods, intermittent fasting has gained popularity due to its flexibility and numerous health benefits. This chapter delves into the concept of intermittent fasting, its benefits for yogis, practical implementation strategies, and the scientific basis supporting this ancient practice.

The concept of intermittent fasting

Intermittent fasting (IF) is an eating pattern that alternates between periods of fasting and eating. Unlike traditional diets that focus on what to eat, intermittent fasting focuses on when to eat. There are several methods of intermittent fasting, each with its own fasting and eating windows:

1. **16/8 Method**: This method involves fasting for 16 hours and eating during an 8-hour window. For example, you might eat between 12 PM and 8 PM and fast from 8 PM to 12 PM the next day.

2. **5:2 Diet**: In this approach, you eat normally for five days of the week and restrict your calorie intake to 500-600 calories on the remaining two days.

3. **Eat-Stop-Eat**: This method involves fasting for a full 24 hours once or twice a week.

4. **Alternate-Day Fasting**: This involves alternating between days of normal eating and days of fasting or consuming very few calories.

The underlying principle of intermittent fasting is to give the body regular breaks from food intake, allowing it to undergo various regenerative processes.

Benefits of intermittent fasting for yogis

Intermittent fasting offers numerous benefits that align well with the principles of yoga, enhancing both physical health and spiritual practice.

Physical benefits

1. **Detoxification**: Fasting allows the body to cleanse itself by promoting autophagy, a process where cells remove damaged components and regenerate new ones. This helps in detoxifying the body and improving cellular health .

2. **Improved digestion**: Regular fasting periods give the digestive system a break, allowing it to reset and function more efficiently. This can lead to better nutrient absorption and reduced digestive issues such as bloating and constipation .

3. **Enhanced metabolism**: Intermittent fasting can boost metabolism by increasing levels of norepinephrine, a hormone that helps burn fat. This can aid in weight management and improve overall metabolic health.

4. **Increased Energy Levels**: Many people report feeling more energetic and focused during fasting periods. This is partly due to the stabilization of blood sugar levels and the reduction in insulin spikes that come with regular eating.

Mental and emotional benefits

1. **Mental clarity**: Fasting promotes mental clarity and focus by reducing oxidative stress and inflammation in the brain. This can enhance cognitive function and improve concentration, which is beneficial for meditation and other mental practices.

2. **Emotional stability**: Regular fasting can help regulate mood swings and reduce symptoms of anxiety and depression. This is linked to the balancing effects of fasting on hormones such as serotonin and dopamine.

Spiritual benefits

1. **Enhanced Meditation**: The mental clarity and focus achieved through fasting can deepen meditation practices, allowing for a more profound spiritual experience. Fasting can also heighten awareness and mindfulness, key components of yoga and meditation.

2. **Discipline and Self-Control**: Fasting requires discipline and self-control, qualities that are essential for a dedicated yoga practice. The practice of fasting can help build these traits, contributing to personal growth and spiritual development.

How to implement intermittent fasting

Implementing intermittent fasting in your lifestyle requires careful planning and a mindful approach. Here are some practical steps to get started:

· Choose a method

Select a fasting method that suits your lifestyle and goals. The 16/8 method is a popular choice for beginners due to its simplicity and flexibility. Start with a method that feels manageable and gradually increase the fasting periods as your body adapts.

· Stay hydrated

Hydration is crucial during fasting periods. Drink plenty of water, herbal teas, and other non-caloric beverages to stay hydrated. This helps maintain energy levels and supports the detoxification process.

· Eat nutrient-dense foods

During eating windows, focus on consuming nutrient-dense, sattvic foods that provide essential vitamins, minerals, and antioxidants. Avoid processed foods, refined sugars, and excessive amounts of caffeine, which can counteract the benefits of fasting.

· **Listen to your body**

Pay attention to how your body responds to fasting. If you feel overly fatigued, dizzy, or unwell, adjust your fasting schedule or consult a healthcare professional. Intermittent fasting should enhance your well-being, not compromise it.

· **Combine with yoga practice**

Incorporate yoga and meditation into your fasting routine to enhance the physical, mental, and spiritual benefits. Gentle yoga practices, such as Hatha or Yin yoga, are particularly beneficial during fasting periods as they promote relaxation and mindfulness.

Scientific basis and traditional wisdom

Intermittent fasting is supported by both modern scientific research and traditional wisdom. Here's a look at how both perspectives converge to validate the benefits of this practice:

Scientific basis

Autophagy and cellular health: Research has shown that intermittent fasting promotes autophagy, a process that helps remove damaged cells and regenerate new ones. This has significant implications for longevity and disease prevention .

Hormonal balance: Intermittent fasting can improve insulin sensitivity and regulate hormones involved in hunger and satiety, such as ghrelin and leptin. This hormonal balance supports weight management and metabolic health .

Brain health: Studies indicate that intermittent fasting can enhance brain function by reducing oxidative stress, inflammation, and promoting neurogenesis (the growth of new brain cells). This can help protect against neurodegenerative diseases and improve cognitive performance .

Traditional wisdom

Ayurveda and fasting: In Ayurvedic tradition, fasting is seen as a way to balance the doshas (body energies) and remove toxins (ama) from the body. It is considered a rejuvenating practice that supports overall health and spiritual growth .

Yogic texts: Ancient yogic texts, such as the Upanishads and the Bhagavad Gita, mention fasting as a means of purification and self-discipline. These texts highlight the importance of fasting for spiritual development and maintaining a clear, focused mind (yogajala) (Fitsri Yoga).

Cultural practices: Fasting has been practiced for centuries in various cultures and religions, often as a means of achieving spiritual clarity and physical detoxification. The convergence of these traditional practices with modern scientific understanding underscores the holistic benefits of intermittent fasting.

By understanding and implementing intermittent fasting, you can harness the power of this ancient practice to enhance your physical health, mental clarity, and spiritual growth. The next sections will explore one-day fasting, the tradition of Ekadashi, and Epsom salt cleansing, providing further insights into the fasting practices in the yogic tradition.

One-day fasting

One-day fasting, a powerful practice in the yogic tradition, offers numerous benefits for physical health, mental clarity, and spiritual growth. Known as Ekadashi in Hindu culture, this practice is deeply rooted in spiritual rituals and has been embraced by yogis for centuries.

The tradition of Ekadashi (fasting day)

Ekadashi, which translates to "the eleventh day," occurs twice a month on the eleventh day of each lunar fortnight in the Hindu calendar. It is considered a highly auspicious day for fasting and spiritual activities. According to Vedic texts, Ekadashi fasting helps to purify the body and mind, removing negative influences and promoting spiritual growth.

Historical and cultural significance

Ekadashi fasting is mentioned in various ancient scriptures, including the Puranas and the Bhagavad Gita. It is believed that observing this fast with devotion and sincerity brings numerous benefits, such as cleansing the body of toxins, improving mental clarity, and aiding in spiritual progress. The tradition of Ekadashi has been passed down through generations, with millions of practitioners observing the fast to this day.

Spiritual practices on Ekadashi

On Ekadashi, devotees often engage in spiritual practices such as prayer, meditation, and reading sacred texts. The day is dedicated to introspection, self-discipline, and connecting with the divine. Abstaining from food and certain activities is seen as a way to conserve energy and focus on spiritual pursuits.

Benefits of one day fasting

One-day fasting, particularly on Ekadashi, offers a range of benefits that enhance physical, mental, and spiritual well-being.

Physical benefits

1. **Detoxification**: Fasting gives the digestive system a break, allowing the body to eliminate accumulated toxins. This detoxification process supports liver function and overall health.

2. **Improved digestion**: By abstaining from food for a day, the digestive system can rest and reset, leading to better digestion and nutrient absorption in the following days.

3. **Weight management**: Regular one-day fasting can help maintain a healthy weight by promoting fat metabolism and reducing calorie intake.

4. **Enhanced immunity**: Fasting has been shown to boost the immune system by reducing inflammation and improving the body's ability to fight infections.

Mental benefits

1. **Increased mental clarity**: Fasting helps clear mental fog and improves focus and concentration. The reduction in food intake allows the brain to function more efficiently.

2. **Emotional stability**: One-day fasting can help stabilize emotions by reducing stress and anxiety. The practice encourages mindfulness and emotional resilience.

3. **Better sleep**: Many practitioners report improved sleep quality following a day of fasting, as the body and mind are more relaxed.

Spiritual benefits

1. **Deeper meditation**: Fasting enhances the ability to meditate deeply by promoting mental calmness and focus. The absence of digestive activity allows more energy to be directed toward spiritual practices.

2. **Heightened awareness**: One-day fasting increases awareness and mindfulness, making it easier to connect with one's inner self and the divine.

3. **Spiritual growth**: Regular fasting helps develop self-discipline, willpower, and a deeper sense of devotion, all of which are essential for spiritual growth.

Practical guidelines for a successful fast

To reap the full benefits of one-day fasting, it is important to follow certain guidelines and prepare adequately.

Preparation

1. **Light meals before fasting**: Consume light, sattvic meals the day before the fast. Avoid heavy, spicy, and tamasic foods that can burden the digestive system.

2. **Hydration**: Ensure you are well-hydrated before starting the fast. Drink plenty of water and herbal teas to prepare your body for the fasting period.

During the fast

1. **Stay hydrated**: Drink water, coconut water, and herbal teas throughout the fasting day to stay hydrated and support detoxification.

2. **Engage in spiritual practices**: Use the fasting day for meditation, prayer, and reading sacred texts. Engage in activities that promote inner peace and spiritual growth.

3. **Rest and relax**: Avoid strenuous physical activities and allow your body to rest. Gentle yoga and breathing exercises can be beneficial.

Breaking the fast

1. **Light foods**: Break your fast with light, easily digestible foods such as fruits, vegetable soups, and smoothies. Gradually reintroduce solid foods to avoid overwhelming the digestive system.

2. **Mindful eating**: Eat slowly and mindfully, paying attention to your body's hunger signals and avoiding overeating.

Testimonials and case studies

Numerous individuals have experienced profound benefits from one-day fasting, particularly on Ekadashi. Here are a few testimonials and case studies that highlight the transformative power of this practice:

Testimonial 1: Enhanced mental clarity and focus

A seasoned yoga practitioner shares how one-day fasting on Ekadashi has improved their mental clarity and focus. "Fasting on Ekadashi has become a crucial part of my routine. It clears my mind, enhances my meditation, and makes me feel more connected to my spiritual path."

Testimonial 2: Improved digestion and overall health

A health enthusiast recounts their journey with one-day fasting: "Initially, I started fasting to manage my weight, but the benefits went far beyond that. My digestion has improved significantly, and I feel more energetic and healthy overall."

Case Study: Spiritual growth and emotional stability

A case study of a yoga teacher who incorporates Ekadashi fasting into their practice reveals remarkable improvements in emotional stability and spiritual growth. "Fasting has taught me discipline and patience. It has deepened my spiritual practices and brought a sense of calm and balance into my life."

Conclusion

One-day fasting, particularly on Ekadashi, is a powerful practice that offers a myriad of benefits for the mind, body, and spirit. By understanding the tradition, following practical guidelines, and learning from others' experiences, you can integrate this transformative practice into your yogic lifestyle, enhancing your overall well-being and spiritual growth.

Epsom salt cleansing

Epsom salt, also known as magnesium sulfate, has long been used for its therapeutic properties, particularly in detoxification and cleansing practices. Incorporating Epsom salt into your fasting routine can enhance the detoxification process, supporting both physical and mental well-being. This chapter explores the role of Epsom salt in fasting, practical steps for using it for body cleansing, and essential safety precautions.

The role of epsom salt in fasting

Epsom salt plays a significant role in fasting by facilitating the body's natural detoxification processes. When ingested, Epsom salt acts as a powerful laxative, helping to cleanse the digestive tract and eliminate accumulated toxins. This practice can enhance the benefits of fasting, promoting overall health and vitality.

Benefits of epsom salt in fasting

1. **Detoxification**: Epsom salt helps draw out toxins from the body, supporting liver function and enhancing the body's natural detoxification processes.

2. **Improved digestion**: By acting as a laxative, Epsom salt helps clear the digestive tract, promoting regular bowel movements and improving digestive health.

3. **Increased magnesium levels**: Magnesium is an essential mineral involved in numerous bodily functions, including muscle and nerve function, energy production, and regulation of blood sugar levels. Consuming Epsom salt can help replenish magnesium levels, supporting overall health.

How to use epsom salt for body cleansing

To effectively use Epsom salt for body cleansing, it is crucial to follow specific steps and guidelines. Here's a detailed guide on how to incorporate Epsom salt into your cleansing routine:

Morning routine

1. **Preparation**: Start by measuring 30 grams of Epsom salt (approximately two tablespoons). Ensure the Epsom salt is food-grade to avoid impurities and potential contaminants.

2. **Mixing**: Dissolve the Epsom salt in a full glass of warm water (about 8 ounces). Stir well until the salt is completely dissolved. This helps ensure that the solution is evenly mixed and easier to drink.

3. **Consumption**: Drink the Epsom salt solution first thing in the morning on an empty stomach. The timing is essential to maximize the detoxifying effects and ensure that the digestive system is ready to process the solution effectively.

Post-Consumption effects

1. **Hydration**: After consuming the Epsom salt solution, drink plenty of water to stay hydrated. This helps flush out toxins and supports the body's natural cleansing processes.

2. **Bathroom access**: Within 30 minutes to an hour, you may begin to experience the laxative effects of the Epsom salt. It is normal to have several bowel movements during this time. Stay near a bathroom to ensure comfort and convenience.

3. **Rest and relaxation**: Take it easy during the cleansing process. Rest and avoid strenuous activities to allow your body to focus on detoxification.

Breaking the fast

1. **Light foods**: After the cleansing process, start with light, easily digestible foods such as fruits, vegetable soups, and smoothies. Avoid heavy, greasy, or processed foods that can burden the digestive system.

2. **Gradual reintroduction**: Gradually reintroduce regular foods into your diet over the next day or two. This helps your digestive system adjust and prevents discomfort.

Safety precautions and tips

While Epsom salt cleansing can offer numerous benefits, it is essential to follow safety guidelines to avoid potential risks and ensure a safe and effective cleansing experience.

Consultation

1. **Medical advice**: Always consult with a healthcare provider before starting an Epsom salt cleanse, especially if you have underlying health conditions or are taking medications. Your doctor can provide personalized advice and ensure that the cleanse is safe for you.

2. **Pregnancy and nursing**: Pregnant and nursing women should avoid Epsom salt cleansing unless advised by a healthcare provider. The effects of magnesium sulfate on pregnancy and breastfeeding are not fully understood, so it is best to err on the side of caution.

Dosage and frequency

1. **Correct dosage**: Stick to the recommended dosage of 30 grams (two tablespoons) of Epsom salt dissolved in water. Using more than the recommended amount can lead to adverse effects such as diarrhea, dehydration, and electrolyte imbalances.

2. **Frequency**: Limit Epsom salt cleansing to once a month or as recommended by your healthcare provider. Overuse can disrupt the body's natural balance and lead to potential health issues.

Hydration and nutrition

1. **Stay hydrated**: Drink plenty of water before, during, and after the cleanse to stay hydrated. This helps flush out toxins and prevents dehydration, a common side effect of laxatives.

2. **Balanced diet**: Ensure your diet is balanced and nutrient-rich before and after the cleanse. Consuming a variety of fruits, vegetables, whole grains, and lean proteins supports overall health and enhances the benefits of the cleanse.

Monitoring and adjustments

1. **Listen to Your Body**: Pay attention to how your body responds to the Epsom salt cleanse. If you experience severe discomfort, cramping, or other adverse effects, discontinue use and consult a healthcare provider.

2. **Adjust as Needed**: If the standard dosage is too harsh, consider reducing the amount of Epsom salt or diluting it with more water. Find a balance that works for your body while still providing the cleansing benefits.

By following these guidelines and safety precautions, you can effectively incorporate Epsom salt cleansing into your fasting routine, enhancing the detoxification process and supporting overall health and well-being. The next chapter will explore practical meal plans and recipes that align with the principles of the yogic diet, providing further support for your journey toward holistic wellness.

Part IV: Recipes and Meal Plans

Sattvic Recipes for Everyday

Incorporating sattvic foods into your daily meals can transform your diet and support your overall well-being. This section provides a variety of sattvic recipes for breakfast, lunch, and dinner, along with snacks and beverages. These recipes are designed to be simple, nutritious, and delicious, aligning with the principles of the yogic diet.

Breakfast Ideas

Sattvic Smoothie Bowl

Ingredients:

- 1 banana
- 1 cup spinach
- 1 cup mixed berries (blueberries, strawberries)
- 1 cup almond milk
- 1 tablespoon chia seeds
- 1 tablespoon almond butter

Instructions:

Blend the banana, spinach, mixed berries, and almond milk until smooth.

Pour into a bowl and top with chia seeds and almond butter.

Add additional toppings such as sliced almonds, coconut flakes, or fresh fruit as desired.

Oatmeal with Fresh Fruits and Nuts

Ingredients:

1 cup rolled oats

2 cups water or almond milk

1 apple, diced

1 teaspoon cinnamon

1 tablespoon almond butter

1 tablespoon chia seeds

A handful of fresh berries (blueberries, raspberries)

Instructions:

Cook the oats in water or almond milk according to package instructions.

Stir in the diced apple and cinnamon.

Serve topped with almond butter, chia seeds, and fresh berries.

Sources: Yoga Journal and Mindbodygreen

Lunch and dinner recipes

Quinoa and vegetable salad

Ingredients:

1 cup quinoa

2 cups water

1 cucumber, diced

1 bell pepper, diced

1 cup cherry tomatoes, halved

1/4 cup red onion, finely chopped

1/4 cup parsley, chopped

2 tablespoons olive oil

1 lemon, juiced

Salt and pepper to taste

Instructions:

Rinse the quinoa under cold water. Combine quinoa and water in a pot and bring to a boil. Reduce heat and simmer for 15 minutes or until water is absorbed. Let cool.

In a large bowl, combine the cooked quinoa, cucumber, bell pepper, cherry tomatoes, red onion, and parsley.

Drizzle with olive oil and lemon juice, and season with salt and pepper. Toss to combine.

Lentil and spinach soup

Ingredients:

1 cup lentils

6 cups vegetable broth

1 onion, diced

2 cloves garlic, minced

2 carrots, diced

2 celery stalks, diced

2 cups fresh spinach

1 teaspoon cumin

1 teaspoon turmeric

Salt and pepper to taste

Instructions:

In a large pot, sauté the onion and garlic until fragrant.

Add the carrots and celery, and cook for a few more minutes.

Add the lentils, vegetable broth, cumin, turmeric, salt, and pepper. Bring to a boil, then reduce heat and simmer for 30 minutes.

Stir in the spinach and cook until wilted. Adjust seasoning as needed.

Fresh fruit salad

Ingredients:

  1 cup pineapple, diced

  1 cup mango, diced

  1 cup blueberries

  1 cup strawberries, sliced

  Juice of 1 lime

  Fresh mint leaves, chopped

Instructions:

  Combine all the fruit in a large bowl.

  Drizzle with lime juice and sprinkle with chopped mint.

  Toss gently to combine and serve chilled.

Almond and date energy balls

Ingredients:

  1 cup almonds

  1 cup pitted dates

  2 tablespoons cocoa powder

  1 tablespoon coconut oil

  1 teaspoon vanilla extract

Instructions:

In a food processor, blend the almonds until finely ground.

Add the dates, cocoa powder, coconut oil, and vanilla extract. Blend until the mixture forms a sticky dough.

Roll the mixture into small balls and refrigerate for at least 30 minutes before serving.

Herbal tea blend

Ingredients:

1 teaspoon dried chamomile

1 teaspoon dried lavender

1 teaspoon dried peppermint

2 cups boiling water

Instructions:

Combine the dried herbs in a teapot or infuser.

Pour boiling water over the herbs and steep for 5-10 minutes.

Strain and serve warm.

By incorporating these sattvic recipes into your daily meal plans, you can enjoy a variety of delicious and nutritious foods that support your physical health, mental clarity, and spiritual growth. These recipes are designed to be easy to prepare, using fresh and wholesome ingredients that align with the principles of the yogic diet.

Fasting friendly recipes

Light meals for intermittent fasting

Intermittent fasting involves alternating periods of eating and fasting. During eating windows, it is essential to consume nutrient-dense, light meals that support your body without overwhelming the digestive system. Here are some light meals that are perfect for intermittent fasting:

Vegetable stir-fry with tofu

Ingredients:

- 1 block firm tofu, cubed
- 2 tablespoons sesame oil
- 1 broccoli head, cut into florets
- 1 red bell pepper, sliced
- 1 carrot, julienned
- 2 cloves garlic, minced
- 1 tablespoon soy sauce (or tamari for gluten-free)
- 1 teaspoon grated ginger
- 1 tablespoon sesame seeds

Instructions:

Heat the sesame oil in a large pan over medium heat.

Add the tofu cubes and cook until golden brown on all sides. Remove and set aside.

In the same pan, add the garlic and ginger, and sauté until fragrant.

Add the broccoli, bell pepper, and carrot, and stir-fry for 5-7 minutes until tender-crisp.

Return the tofu to the pan, add soy sauce, and stir to combine.

Sprinkle with sesame seeds before serving.

Detox soup

Ingredients:

1 onion, diced

2 cloves garlic, minced

1 zucchini, diced

2 carrots, diced

2 celery stalks, diced

1 cup kale, chopped

1 can diced tomatoes

4 cups vegetable broth

1 teaspoon turmeric

1 teaspoon cumin

Salt and pepper to taste

Juice of 1 lemon

Instructions:

In a large pot, sauté the onion and garlic until translucent.

Add the zucchini, carrots, and celery, and cook for a few more minutes.

Stir in the diced tomatoes, vegetable broth, turmeric, cumin, salt, and pepper.

Bring to a boil, then reduce heat and simmer for 20 minutes.

Add the kale and cook for another 5 minutes.

Stir in lemon juice before serving.

Recipes for one day fasting

One-day fasting, particularly on Ekadashi, involves abstaining from food for 24 hours. However, it is important to prepare for and break the fast with light, easily digestible meals to support your body. Here are some recipes suitable for the day before and after the fast:

Pre-fast light meal: Quinoa and vegetable stew

Ingredients:

1 cup quinoa, rinsed

2 cups water

1 zucchini, diced

1 carrot, diced

1 celery stalk, diced

1 tomato, chopped

1 cup spinach, chopped

2 tablespoons olive oil

1 teaspoon cumin

Salt and pepper to taste

Instructions:

In a pot, bring the quinoa and water to a boil. Reduce heat and simmer for 15 minutes until the water is absorbed.

In a separate pan, heat the olive oil and sauté the zucchini, carrot, and celery until tender.

Add the tomato, spinach, cumin, salt, and pepper, and cook until the vegetables are softened.

Stir in the cooked quinoa and combine well.

Post-fast light meal: Mango lassi

Ingredients:

1 ripe mango, peeled and chopped

1 cup plain yogurt

1/2 cup water

1 tablespoon honey (optional)

1/4 teaspoon ground cardamom

Instructions:

In a blender, combine the mango, yogurt, water, honey (if using), and cardamom.

Blend until smooth.

Serve chilled.

Simple fruit and nut salad

Ingredients:

1 apple, diced

1 banana, sliced

1/2 cup grapes, halved

1/4 cup walnuts, chopped

1 tablespoon honey

Juice of 1/2 lemon

Instructions:

Combine the apple, banana, grapes, and walnuts in a bowl.

Drizzle with honey and lemon juice.

Toss gently to combine and serve immediately.

By incorporating these fasting-friendly recipes into your routine, you can support your body's detoxification processes while ensuring you receive essential nutrients. These light, wholesome meals are designed to be easy on the digestive system, making them perfect for intermittent and one-day fasting practices.

Part V: Integrating the yogic diet into daily life

Integrating the yogic diet into your daily life can be a transformative experience, promoting physical health, mental clarity, and spiritual growth. However, like any significant lifestyle change, it comes with its own set of challenges. This section addresses common obstacles and provides practical solutions to help you stay motivated and consistent, while also building a supportive environment.

Overcoming challenges

Adopting a yogic diet may present several challenges, particularly if you are transitioning from a more conventional diet. Here are some common challenges and strategies to overcome them:

Time management

Challenge: Finding the time to prepare fresh, sattvic meals can be difficult, especially with a busy schedule.

Solution: Plan and prepare meals in advance. Batch cooking and meal prepping can save time and ensure you always have healthy options available. Set aside a few hours each week to cook and store meals in the refrigerator or freezer. Use simple recipes that require minimal preparation but still provide balanced nutrition.

Social situations

Challenge: Navigating social events and dining out can be challenging when adhering to a yogic diet.

Solution: Communicate your dietary preferences in advance. When attending social gatherings, offer to bring a dish that aligns with your diet. Research restaurant menus ahead of time to find suitable options or request modifications to meet your dietary needs.

Cravings and temptations

Challenge: Dealing with cravings for rajasic or tamasic foods can be difficult, especially during the initial transition.

Solution: Gradually reduce the intake of non-sattvic foods rather than eliminating them all at once. Find healthy, sattvic alternatives to your favorite foods. For example, replace sugary snacks with fresh fruits or nuts. Practice mindful eating to recognize and manage cravings.

Common obstacles and solutions

Limited access to fresh produce

Obstacle: Access to fresh, organic produce can be limited in some areas.

Solution: Shop at local farmers' markets or join a community-supported agriculture (CSA) program to get fresh, seasonal produce. Grow your own vegetables and herbs if you have space. When fresh produce is not available, opt for frozen fruits and vegetables, which retain most of their nutrients.

Nutritional concerns

Obstacle: Ensuring you get all the essential nutrients on a vegetarian or vegan yogic diet.

Solution: Eat a variety of fruits, vegetables, whole grains, legumes, nuts, and seeds to cover all nutrient bases. Consider supplements for nutrients that might be harder to obtain from a plant-based diet, such as vitamin B12, vitamin D, and omega-3 fatty acids. Consult a nutritionist or dietitian if needed.

Staying motivated and consistent

Maintaining motivation and consistency is key to successfully integrating the yogic diet into your life. Here are some strategies to help you stay on track:

Set clear goals

Define your reasons for adopting the yogic diet, whether for health, spiritual growth, or ethical considerations. Having clear goals will help you stay focused and motivated.

Track your progress

Keep a journal to track your meals, how you feel physically and mentally, and any challenges you encounter. Reflecting on your progress can provide motivation and highlight the benefits you're experiencing.

Celebrate small wins

Acknowledge and celebrate your successes, no matter how small. Whether it's trying a new recipe, sticking to your diet during a challenging week, or feeling more energized, recognizing these milestones can boost your motivation.

Stay educated

Continuously educate yourself about the benefits of the yogic diet and explore new recipes and cooking techniques. Reading books, attending workshops, and joining online communities can keep you inspired and informed.

Building a supportive environment

Creating a supportive environment is crucial for sustaining dietary changes. Here are some tips for building a supportive network:

Involve family and friends

Share your journey with family and friends. Explain the benefits of the yogic diet and invite them to try it with you. Having a support system can make the transition easier and more enjoyable.

Join a community

Join local or online communities focused on yoga and sattvic living. These communities can provide encouragement, share experiences, and offer valuable tips and recipes.

Create a conducive home environment

Stock your kitchen with sattvic foods and cooking tools that make meal preparation easier. Remove or minimize non-sattvic foods to reduce temptation. Create a peaceful dining area that encourages mindful eating.

By addressing these challenges with practical solutions and maintaining a positive, flexible approach, you can successfully integrate the yogic diet into your daily life. This holistic approach to eating not only nourishes your body but also enhances mental clarity and spiritual growth, leading to a balanced and fulfilling life.

Personal Stories and Testimonials

Experiences from practitioners

Integrating the yogic diet into one's life is a deeply personal journey that can lead to profound transformations in health, mental clarity, and spiritual growth. Here, we share personal stories and testimonials from practitioners who have embraced the yogic diet and experienced its benefits firsthand.

Testimonial 1: Finding balance and peace

Name: Sarah Thompson
Age: 34
Occupation: Yoga Instructor

Her story:

Sarah Thompson, a dedicated yoga instructor, began her journey with the yogic diet five years ago. Struggling with digestive issues and chronic fatigue, she sought a holistic approach to healing that aligned with her yoga practice.

"I was constantly feeling bloated and tired, and my energy levels were inconsistent. A fellow yoga teacher introduced me to the concept of sattvic foods and the yogic diet. I started incorporating more fresh fruits, vegetables, whole grains, and reducing my intake of processed foods and caffeine," Sarah recalls.

Impact:

The changes were almost immediate. Sarah noticed improved digestion, sustained energy levels, and a greater sense of inner peace. Her meditation practices deepened, and she felt more connected to her spiritual path.

"Adopting the yogic diet has been a game-changer for me. Not only did my physical health improve, but I also felt more mentally and spiritually balanced. It's a lifestyle that truly aligns with my values and my practice."

Testimonial 2: Overcoming emotional eating

Name: Michael Rodriguez
Age: 45
Occupation: Corporate Executive

His story:

Michael Rodriguez, a corporate executive with a demanding job, turned to the yogic diet to manage stress and emotional eating. His high-stress job often led to unhealthy eating habits and weight gain, impacting his overall well-being.

"I was trapped in a cycle of stress and emotional eating, which was affecting my health and my ability to focus at work. I decided to try the yogic diet after reading about its benefits for mental clarity and emotional balance," Michael explains.

Impact:

Michael started with simple changes, like replacing processed snacks with fresh fruits and practicing mindful eating. Over time, he transitioned to a fully sattvic diet.

"The results were remarkable. Not only did I lose weight, but I also felt more centered and less reactive to stress. The yogic diet helped me develop a healthier relationship with food and brought a sense of calm and focus to my hectic life."

Testimonial 3: Enhancing spiritual practices

Name: Anjali Patel
Age: 28
Occupation: Artist

Her story:

Anjali Patel, an artist and avid yoga practitioner, embraced the yogic diet to enhance her spiritual practices. She felt that her diet was not supporting her spiritual aspirations and sought a deeper connection with her inner self.

"I wanted my diet to reflect my spiritual journey and support my yoga and meditation practices. The yogic diet seemed like the perfect fit, emphasizing purity, balance, and mindfulness," says Anjali.

Impact:

By incorporating sattvic foods and practicing mindful eating, Anjali experienced a profound transformation in her spiritual practices. Her meditation sessions became deeper and more fulfilling, and she felt a stronger sense of spiritual connection.

"The yogic diet has been incredibly transformative for my spiritual journey. It has brought a new level of clarity and peace to my life, and I feel more aligned with my true self."

The transformative power of the yogic diet

The yogic diet has the potential to transform lives by promoting holistic well-being. Here are some key aspects of its transformative power:

Physical Transformation

Improved Health:

The yogic diet emphasizes natural, unprocessed foods rich in nutrients, which support overall health. Practitioners often report better digestion, increased energy, weight management, and enhanced immunity.

Detoxification:

The diet's focus on fresh fruits, vegetables, and whole grains aids in detoxifying the body, removing toxins and promoting optimal organ function.

Mental transformation

Mental clarity:

By reducing the intake of stimulating and heavy foods, the yogic diet helps clear mental fog and enhances concentration and focus. This mental clarity is beneficial for both professional and personal pursuits.

Emotional Balance:

The calming effects of sattvic foods help stabilize emotions, reduce anxiety, and promote a sense of inner peace. Practitioners often feel more resilient and better equipped to handle stress.

Spiritual transformation

Deeper meditation:

A sattvic diet supports deeper and more effective meditation practices. The purity and lightness of these foods align with spiritual goals, enhancing the overall meditation experience.

Spiritual growth:

The principles of the yogic diet—such as mindfulness, gratitude, and purity—foster spiritual growth. Practitioners often report a stronger connection to their higher self and the universe.

By sharing these personal stories and highlighting the transformative power of the yogic diet, it becomes clear that this holistic approach to nutrition can significantly enhance one's physical, mental, and spiritual well-being. Adopting the yogic diet is not just about changing what you eat; it's about embracing a lifestyle that nurtures every aspect of your being.

Bonus: Dietary advice from my guru

Adopting a yogic diet and lifestyle can be transformative, promoting physical health, mental clarity, and spiritual growth. My guru, a seasoned practitioner and teacher of yoga, provided me with invaluable insights and guidelines to enhance the benefits of the yogic diet. Here are some tips and recommendations based on his wisdom:

What can be eaten and what should be avoided

Foods to eat

- **Sattvic Foods**: Fresh fruits and vegetables, whole grains, legumes, nuts, seeds, and dairy products (such as milk and yogurt). Plant-based dairy alternatives (such as almond milk or coconut milk) can also be used.

- **Vegetarian Foods**: Include a variety of vegetables, whole grains (such as brown rice, quinoa, and oats), legumes (such as lentils and chickpeas), and nuts and seeds.

- **Fruits**: All types of fresh fruits are recommended, especially those in season.

Foods to avoid

- **Tamasic Foods**: Meat, fish, eggs, alcohol, and heavily processed foods.

- **Rajasic Foods**: Excessively spicy foods, caffeine (coffee and tea), chocolate, and foods with artificial additives and preservatives.

Note for Meat Eaters: If you still eat meat, try to reduce consumption to once a week, preferably on Sundays. Avoid red meat and choose chicken or turkey instead.

Other Substances to Avoid: Smoking, drinking alcohol, and the use of drugs should be avoided to maintain the purity and balance of mind and body.

Weekly Example Diet Plans

Weight Loss Plan

Monday: Fasting (optional epsom salt cleanse)

Tuesday: Vegetarian food

Wednesday: Vegetarian food

Thursday: Only fruits
(or fasting with epsom salt cleanse for faster results)

Friday: Rice day

    Breakfast/Lunch: Rice pudding

    Dinner: Rice with vegetables

Saturday: Vegetarian food

Sunday: Vegetarian food (or chicken/turkey for meat eaters)

Weight Maintenance Plan

Monday: Fasting (optional Epsom salt cleanse)

Tuesday: Vegetarian food

Wednesday: Vegetarian food

Thursday: Only fruits

Friday: Vegetarian food

Saturday: Vegetarian food

Sunday: Vegetarian food (or chicken/turkey for meat
eaters)

Note:
*When the desired weight is achieved, the Epsom salt cleanse
can be done every two weeks or once a month. 30 minutes
before each meal, eat two fruits. If not possible, wait at least 5
minutes after eating the fruit. No food or snacking between
meals, and no food after 21:00. Try not to overeat and fill*

your stomach to 80 percent to leave room for water and air. Drinking water a little after meals is okay, but not too much because it will dilute the stomach juices. Try to drink 30-40 minutes after food intake. The start of the week and fasting days can be adjusted to your preference. For example, you might fast on Wednesday, eat fruit on Saturday, and have a rice day on Sunday.

Fasting and epsom salt cleanse

Fasting guidelines:
On fasting days, drink plenty of water. If you are new to fasting, you may drink milk to help with hunger, in addition to water.

Epsom salt cleanse instructions:

- In the morning, dissolve 30 grams of Epsom salt in a glass of water and drink it.
- 10-15 minutes aft the first visit to the toilet, drink a glass of room temperature milk.

Choosing the right day for epsom salt cleanse

When planning an Epsom salt cleanse, choose your day carefully as the process can take up the entire day several visits to the bathroom. It's best to select a day when you have no other commitments, allowing you to stay home and rest as needed.

These guidelines from my guru provide a structured approach to integrating the yogic diet into your daily life. By following this regimen, you can experience the profound benefits of the yogic diet, including improved health, mental clarity, and spiritual growth. Remember, consistency and mindfulness in your dietary practices are key to achieving and maintaining holistic well-being.

By following these simple guidelines and the weekly diet plan, you can achieve your health goals while embracing the principles of the yogic diet. This approach not only helps in weight management but also promotes overall well-being, clarity of mind, and spiritual growth. Enjoy your journey towards a healthier, more balanced life.

Conclusion

Embracing a yogic diet for life

Embracing a yogic diet is not just about making temporary changes to your eating habits; it is about adopting a holistic lifestyle that fosters physical health, mental clarity, and spiritual growth. The principles of the yogic diet are deeply rooted in ancient traditions and provide a framework for living a balanced and harmonious life. By integrating these principles into your daily routine, you can experience profound and lasting benefits.

Long-term benefits

The long-term benefits of adhering to a yogic diet are extensive and multifaceted, impacting every aspect of your being.

Physical health

Improved digestion: A diet rich in sattvic foods supports healthy digestion and regular bowel movements, reducing digestive issues such as bloating and constipation.

Enhanced immunity: The nutrients and antioxidants found in fresh fruits, vegetables, and whole grains strengthen the immune system, helping the body fight off infections and illnesses.

Sustained energy levels: Sattvic foods provide steady, sustained energy throughout the day, avoiding the peaks and crashes associated with processed and sugary foods.

Weight Management: The natural, nutrient-dense foods of the yogic diet support healthy weight management without the need for restrictive dieting.

Mental clarity

Increased focus: The yogic diet promotes mental clarity and concentration, essential for effective meditation and mindfulness practices.

Emotional stability: A diet rich in sattvic foods helps stabilize mood swings and reduces anxiety and stress, promoting emotional resilience.

Better sleep: The calming effects of sattvic foods contribute to improved sleep quality and regular sleep patterns.

Spiritual growth

Deepened meditation: A sattvic diet supports deeper, more effective meditation by promoting mental calmness and focus.

Enhanced mindfulness: Mindful eating practices foster a greater connection with food, cultivating gratitude and awareness in everyday life.

Spiritual connection: By aligning your diet with the principles of sattva, you cultivate a lifestyle that supports your spiritual journey and deepens your connection to your higher self and the universe.

Continuing your journey

The journey of adopting and maintaining a yogic diet is ongoing and ever-evolving. It requires commitment, mindfulness, and a willingness to explore and adapt. Here are some tips for continuing your journey:

Stay informed

Continuously educate yourself about the benefits of the yogic diet and explore new recipes, cooking techniques, and nutritional insights. Stay updated with the latest research and integrate new knowledge into your dietary practices.

Be flexible

While it is important to adhere to the principles of the yogic diet, it is also essential to remain flexible and adaptable. Life circumstances, social situations, and personal preferences may require adjustments. Embrace these changes with a positive attitude and find ways to stay aligned with your dietary goals.

Practice mindfulness

Mindfulness is a cornerstone of the yogic diet. Practice mindful eating by being fully present during meals, savoring each bite, and appreciating the food's journey from nature to your plate. This practice enhances digestion, deepens your connection with food, and promotes overall well-being.

Encouragement for ongoing exploration

The yogic diet is a journey of exploration and self-discovery. Here are some final words of encouragement as you continue on this path:

Embrace the journey

Remember that adopting a yogic diet is a journey, not a destination. Embrace each step with curiosity and openness, and celebrate your progress along the way. Every small change and mindful choice contributes to your overall well-being.

Connect with community

Join local or online communities of like-minded individuals who are also exploring the yogic diet. Sharing experiences, tips, and recipes can provide valuable support and inspiration.

Keep Exploring

Continue to explore new foods, recipes, and dietary practices that align with the principles of the yogic diet. Experiment with different fasting techniques, meal plans, and mindfulness practices to find what works best for you.

By embracing the yogic diet and incorporating its principles into your daily life, you can cultivate a balanced, healthy, and spiritually fulfilling lifestyle. The journey is ongoing, and each day offers new opportunities for growth and transformation. Stay committed, stay mindful, and enjoy the profound benefits of the yogic diet.

With these insights and tips, you are well-equipped to embrace the yogic diet for life. May your journey be filled with health, clarity, and spiritual growth.

Appendices

Glossary of Terms

Ahimsa: A principle of non-violence toward all living beings, central to yogic philosophy and practice.

Asana: A physical posture or pose in yoga, designed to enhance strength, flexibility, and balance.

Ayurveda: An ancient Indian system of medicine that focuses on balance and harmony between the body, mind, and spirit through diet, lifestyle, and herbal remedies.

Dosha: In Ayurveda, the three energies (Vata, Pitta, and Kapha) believed to govern physical and mental processes.

Ekadashi: The eleventh day of each lunar fortnight in the Hindu calendar, considered an auspicious day for fasting and spiritual activities.

Prana: The vital life force or energy that sustains all living beings, often cultivated through breath control (pranayama) in yoga.

Pranayama: The practice of breath control in yoga, aimed at enhancing prana and promoting physical and mental well-being.

Rajasic Foods: Foods that are stimulating and can lead to restlessness and agitation. Examples include spicy foods, caffeine, and processed snacks.

Sattvic Foods: Pure, fresh, and natural foods that promote clarity, calmness, and spiritual growth. Examples include fruits, vegetables, whole grains, and nuts.

Tamasic Foods: Heavy and dull foods that promote lethargy and confusion. Examples include meat, alcohol, and overly processed foods.

Yogic Diet: A dietary approach rooted in the principles of Ayurveda and yoga, emphasizing sattvic foods and mindful eating practices to support physical, mental, and spiritual health.

Sources:
Yoga Journal, Mindbodygreen, The Ayurvedic Institute

Key Terms and Definitions

Detoxification: The process of removing toxins from the body, often supported by dietary practices like fasting and consuming detoxifying foods.

Mindful Eating: A practice of eating with full attention and awareness, focusing on the sensory experience of food and recognizing hunger and satiety cues.

Intermittent Fasting: An eating pattern that alternates between periods of fasting and eating, promoting detoxification and various health benefits.

Autophagy: A cellular process that removes damaged components and regenerates new ones, often enhanced by fasting practices.

Spiritual Growth: The process of deepening one's connection with their inner self and the divine, often facilitated by practices like meditation, yoga, and a sattvic diet.

Sources: Healthline, WebMD, The Chopra Center

Resources and further reading

Recommended books

"The Complete Book of Ayurvedic Home Remedies" by Vasant Lad: A comprehensive guide to using Ayurvedic principles for healing and maintaining health.

"The Yoga of Herbs: An Ayurvedic Guide to Herbal Medicine" by David Frawley and Vasant Lad: An exploration of herbal remedies in the context of Ayurveda and yoga.

"The Heart of Yoga: Developing a Personal Practice" by T.K.V. Desikachar: A foundational text on the principles and practice of yoga, including dietary recommendations.

Sources:

Yoga Journal: Articles and resources on yoga practices, principles, and dietary guidelines.

Mindbodygreen: Articles on holistic health, wellness, and mindful living.

The Chopra Center: Resources on Ayurveda, meditation, and holistic health.

Healthline: Comprehensive health information, including benefits of different dietary practices.

WebMD: Health information and advice on various conditions, treatments, and wellness practices.

The Ayurvedic Institute: Information on Ayurveda, including dietary practices and remedies.

Santosha Yoga Institute: Educational resources on yoga and Ayurvedic principles.

National Center for Complementary and Integrative Health: Research and information on complementary and integrative health practices.

Eat Right: Nutritional advice and guidelines from the Academy of Nutrition and Dietetics.

Wellness Mama: Articles and tips on natural health, wellness, and nutrition.

Nature: Scientific articles and research on health and wellness.

Science Direct: Research articles on various health topics, including intermittent fasting and nutrition.

PubMed Central: Repository of biomedical and life sciences journal literature.

National Institutes of Health (NIH): Health information and research from the U.S. government.

92

Frequently Asked Questions

Addressing Common Concerns

Q: Can I follow a yogic diet if I am not a vegetarian?

A: While the traditional yogic diet emphasizes vegetarianism, it can be adapted to individual needs. The focus should be on consuming predominantly sattvic foods and minimizing tamasic and rajasic foods. If you choose to include animal products, opt for ethically sourced, organic options.

Q: How do I manage social situations while following a yogic diet?

A: Communicate your dietary preferences in advance and offer to bring a dish that aligns with your diet. Research restaurant menus beforehand to find suitable options or request modifications. Practicing mindful eating can also help you stay on track without feeling deprived.

Q: What should I do if I experience cravings for non-sattvic foods?

A: Gradually reduce the intake of non-sattvic foods rather than eliminating them all at once. Find healthy, sattvic alternatives to your favorite foods and practice mindful eating to recognize and manage cravings. Over time, your taste preferences may naturally shift towards more sattvic foods.

Q: Is it necessary to fast to follow a yogic diet?

A: Fasting is a beneficial practice in the yogic tradition, but it is not mandatory. If fasting is difficult, you can start with lighter fasting methods, such as consuming only milk and water on fasting days. Gradually incorporate more fasting practices as you become more comfortable.

I

- Intermittent Fasting
- Improved Digestion

M

- Mental Clarity
- Mindful Eating

N

- Nutrient-Dense Foods
- Nuts and Seeds

P

- Physical Health
- Prana

R

- Rajasic Foods
- Rice Day

S

- Sattvic Foods
- Spiritual Growth

T

- Tamasic Foods
- Traditional Wisdom

Y

- Yogic Diet
- Yogic Lifestyle

By providing these additional resources, definitions, and FAQs, you can enhance your understanding and practice of the yogic diet, ensuring a holistic approach to your health and well-being.